Mediterranean Diet

The Ultimate Guide to Losing Weight Naturally and Feeling Healthy

Mathew Noll

© 2016

responsibility of the recipient reader. Under no circumstances will any legal responsibility or blame be held against the publisher for any reparation, damages, or monetary loss due to the information herein, either directly or indirectly.

Respective authors own all copyrights not held by the publisher.

The information herein is offered for informational purposes solely, and is universal as so. The presentation of the information is without contract or any type of guarantee assurance.

The trademarks that are used are without any consent, and the publication of the trademark is without permission or backing by the trademark owner. All trademarks and brands within this book are for clarifying purposes only and are owned by the owners themselves, not affiliated with this document.

CONTENTS

INTRODUCTION

As opposed to the famous notion, the Mediterranean diet is not just about eating hysterically, even if it is vegetarian food most of the time. If you visit any Mediterranean country, you will not find people eating like the way Americans eat. People living near the sea are very much cautious about what they eat and how much they eat.

The American diet has given such addictive foods to people such as mayonnaise, cheese, packaged chips, sugar filled beverages, creamy meat, etc. These foods are no doubt tasty, but are harmful too. The typical American diet is limited or restricted only for the namesake. In reality, Americans eat larger portions of food than other cultures around the globe. Many people consider a limited diet as healthy if it does not consist of pasta and bread, but a standard diet in America consists of such bland cuisines as the spine of their regular meals.

Now, if you eliminate pasta and bread from your meal and replace them with whole foods, you have to be very creative with your cooking and food preparation. If you do not eat bread, you cannot consume unhealthy sandwiches at lunch. It needs you to instead consume real foods, which demand a slight knowledge of cooking and some efforts in preparation. This is best demonstrated with the standard American breakfast.

Most Americans consume these things at breakfast: muffins, coffee, and cereal. On the other hand, a typical limited breakfast consists of fasting, any kind of bone broth, coffee along with cream, omelet or eggs, and any fermented dairy food. It becomes boring for people to consume the same foods in their breakfast throughout the year, or even for their entire life. Still, they do not want to change or simply do not know how to change. Similarly, lunch also remains the same for years and years; only dinner sees some variation. However, most Americans have started welcoming the change into their diet and they have begun to consume leafy green vegetables in their foods.

The Mediterranean diet gives you a chance to bring positive changes to your life without making much effort. You do not have to be an expert chef to cook Mediterranean meals. There are just a few basic principles of this regime that are very simple to follow. If you are determined to bring back health into your life, you need to be focused about your foods. Go through this book to learn all about the Mediterranean diet and incorporate it practically as soon as possible.

CHAPTER 1

What is the Mediterranean Diet?

Thinking about Mediterranean diet takes most of us to the world of pastas and pizzas of Italy and pita and hummus of Greece. However, this is only half the story; there is much more to the Mediterranean diet than this. The healthier portion of the Mediterranean diet constitutes of fruits, vegetables, hearty grains, olive oil, seafood, and many other things that prepare our body to fight against certain cancers, heart diseases, cognitive decline, and diabetes.

The Mediterranean diet has many benefits that make it worthy of chasing. You can switch from pasta and pepperoni to avocados and fish. You may have to put in significant efforts, but in the end, you will be on your way to a longer as well as healthier life.

What exactly is the Mediterranean diet?
Pizza, gyros, lasagna, falafel, rack of lamb, and white bread long loaves- these foods are synonymous with Mediterranean foods. You might have seen in movies the two hour long, huge feasts with multiple courses as well as endless glasses of wine.

However, the basic idea of the Mediterranean diet is significantly changed because of the addition of unhealthy fats without regard for traditional fruits of the region, nuts, seafood, olive oil, vegetables, beans, red wine, and dairy.

What used to be an inexpensive and healthy way of devouring is now linked with unhealthy, heavy dishes that contribute to obesity, diabetes, heart disease, mood disorders, and many other health ailments. The food pyramid of the Mediterranean diet is based on the dietary traditions of southern Italy, Greece, and Crete of 1960s, the time that saw the lowest rate of unceasing diseases in populations and the life expectancy of adults was one of the highest despite limited medical care. Apart from eating homegrown and fresh foods in place of processed foods, the Mediterranean diet also includes daily exercise, encouraging appreciation for eating delicious and healthy foods, and sharing your food with others.

People of Italy, Spain, Greece, and France are regarded as the healthiest species of humans. These countries are on the borders of the Mediterranean Sea. That is why; the name the Mediterranean diet came into existence. People from these regions have a 30% lower risk of strokes and heart diseases. You can become a Mediterranean person by including these things in your diet:

- Eat plenty of starchy foods like pasta, bread, rice, and potatoes with the skin on to have more fiber.
- Eat fruits and vegetables in abundance, at least 5 portions per day
- Eat less of meat, eggs, pulses, beans, and non- dairy foods
- Eat a small amount of fish
- Eat foods produced from plant oils and vegetables like olive oil
- Have some dairy foods and milk like yoghurt and cheese for calcium and protein.
- Eat less of high fat and high sugar foods

It is better if you make a habit of having Mediterranean foods regularly, but if you cannot follow a strict routine, you can achieve your long- term goals gradually. For instance, you can make weekly goals in place of daily targets. It means that you do not have to 'go on a diet' to follow the Mediterranean diet, but you will be able to lose weight and enhance your well-being. This regime is full of flavor filled, delicious meals, and dishes such as whole grain vegetable pasta, Greek salad, fragrant couscous, creamy hummus and warm pita, and sautéed spinach.

CHAPTER 2

How Does the Mediterranean Diet Do Good to Your Body?

The Mediterranean diet was never meant for losing weight and preventing heart ailments. It evolved naturally with time on the strength of regional foods. Recent researches have proved that Mediterranean diet is capable of improving the way our body deals with insulin and blood sugar. In addition to plenty of healthy fats and omega-3 fatty acids, foods of the Mediterranean diet also give valuable antioxidants that provide immunity against certain types of cancers.

Pros of the Mediterranean diet

Benefits of fruits, vegetables, and seafood are known to everyone. Being a Mediterranean follower, you must know the pros of this diet:

You can follow it for life

The main concern of every person that begins a new diet is whether they will be able to follow it for life or not? The best part about the Mediterranean diet is that you can continue it permanently to stay healthy. The only reason behind sticking with it for life is that you are not on a diet in real sense. You have to just diversify your food.

Low amount of saturated fat

The Mediterranean diet does not consist of low fat foods, but the fat is monounsaturated, which does not raise your level of cholesterol. Saturated fats are present in regular diets and are harmful for heart. Mediterranean foods have healthy fats in the form of fish oil, olive oil, nut-based oil, etc.

Healthy for your heart

Numerous studies have suggested that the followers of the Mediterranean diet face a lower risk of heart ailments than those following a usual American diet.

Prevents cancer

The followers of the Mediterranean diet face a lower risk of prostate, colon cancer, and a few types of neck and head cancer.

Cons of Mediterranean diet

There are not many reasons to be worried about following this diet. However, you need to take care to make sure that you follow these things:

Consume sufficient calcium

The Mediterranean diet is quite short of dairy and milk products, apart from yogurt and cheese. If you are an ardent Mediterranean follower, you must make sure that you consume enough calcium. You can eat more cheese and yogurt or have calcium from non-dairy sources. Many vegetables contain calcium, but if you are fond of milk, you can consume skimmed milk.

Keep a check on wine

The Mediterranean diet emphasizes on red wine, but it does not imply that you can drink overwhelming amounts of it. You should drink only a couple of glasses of wine per day while being aware that an excessive amount of alcohol consumption is linked to breast cancer. It also leads to other kinds of cancers such as oral, esophageal, liver, and laryngeal cancers.

Limit the amount of fat

While the fat contained in Mediterranean foods is healthy, too much of it is obviously not good. Although the Mediterranean diet provides a healthy amount of saturated fat, the total consumption of fat may go overboard if you do not take care.

Learn to cook well

The Mediterranean diet is heavily dependent on your style of cooking. Although you do not have to possess advanced culinary skills, you must improve your cooking abilities with time.

It may be dicey for hyper-sensitive people

You must research a lot about the Mediterranean diet before you begin it. Enlist all the things about this diet that are good or bad for you. If you have a hyper- sensitive body or you are suffering from a health condition, the Mediterranean diet may not be a good option for you.

CHAPTER 3

Does the Mediterranean Diet Really Work?

There is not a particular type of Mediterranean diet. The Greeks have a different eating pattern from the French, who eat unlike the Spanish and the Italians. However, each of these cultures have a common understanding - they all emphasize on eating fruits, whole grains, veggies, beans, nuts, olive oil, legumes, and palatable spices and herbs; eating seafood and fish at least twice a week; eating poultry, cheese, yogurt, and eggs in moderation; and conserving red meat saving sweets for special occasions. Top the foods with a little bit of red wine and stay physically active. It is just so simple to stay fit with a Mediterranean diet.

There is a pattern of eating in this diet since it is not a structured regime. You have to figure it out yourself on how you want to eat and the number of calories you want to maintain or lose weight. You need to figure out your exercising regime and your Mediterranean menu.

The cost of the Mediterranean diet

The Mediterranean diet is a little pricey. Some of the ingredients can be expensive such as olive oil, fresh produce and fish. However, you can buy them cheaply. For instance, you do not have to shell out $50 every time for a wine bottle. You can set a standard to buy a $15 wine bottle. You can buy the vegetables on sale, rather than buying $3 per piece of an artichoke.

How you can lose weight with the Mediterranean diet

If you eat restricted calories in your Mediterranean diet, you can certainly lose weight. It is easy to go overboard with tasty foods, but if you create a calorie deficit in the plan by burning more calories than eating, you can lose weight. As stated earlier, this diet is not designed to lose weight, but can keep you away from being obese or overweight. How quickly you shed your pounds depends on you.

Is it easy to follow the Mediterranean diet?

Since the Mediterranean diet does not ban the whole groups of foods, it is absolutely easy to comply with it in the long-term.

Convenience

If you wish to cook something, there are easy recipes along with complementary wine, which will take you to the ambience of the Atlantic. The consumer friendly pointers will make prepping and meal planning easier. You can eat out as well.

Recipes

The recipes of the Mediterranean diet are simple and most of them cost under $2-$3 for a serving. You can Google the recipes and you will find hundreds of them matching your needs and budget.

Eating out

The Mediterranean diet emphasizes on sharing the meal and embraces the idea of portioning a meal. You can take a friend along when you go to eat out and order a single entrée for both of you. You must ensure that you have some salad and order additional veggies in your meal.

Alcohol

You can consult your doctor before you begin drinking wine on a regular basis. Women can have a glass per day and men can have two glasses daily. The reason behind the popularity of red wine is the presence of resveratrol in it, a compound that prolongs your age. However, drinking wine for all your life will make the difference.

Time saving

You do not have any scope of timesaving if you plan to do all the buying and cooking on your own. You must be ready to invest a part of your day cooking.

Fullness

The experts of nutrition emphasize the worth of fullness, the feeling of being satisfied that you have eaten enough. The Mediterranean diet does not keep you hungry since you have sufficient fiber from the veggies and whole grains.

Taste

Since you cook everything in this diet personally, you can alter the ingredients if you do not like something.

Exercise

You need to exercise daily to burn the calories of Mediterranean foods. You can begin with walking, but add more to it such as jazzercise, pilates, or gardening. You can incorporate anything that you can continue for life. Adults are encouraged to exercise 2.5 hours a week in addition to muscle strengthening exercises on some days.

CHAPTER 4

What You Should Eat in the Mediterranean Diet

The Mediterranean diet dates backs to the foods people used to eat in 1960s. Because of the exceptional health of the Greek and the Italians, they had lower chances of killer diseases. This diet can save you from severe ailments like heart attacks, type 2 diabetes, strokes, premature death, etc.

Diet plan of the Mediterranean diet

We cannot specify a certain way of following the Mediterranean diet. All Mediterranean countries eat different foods. Therefore, you can make a few changes to the different foods mentioned below according to your preferences and needs.

Basics of Mediterranean foods

You must keep in mind a few basic things if you do not want to remember the complex details of the complete food list.

Eat as much as you want

Vegetables, nuts, fruits, seeds, potatoes, legumes, whole grains, spices, breads, herbs, fish, extra virgin olive oil, and seafood.

Eat in temperance

Poultry, eggs, yogurt, and cheese

Eat rarely

Red meat

Keep away from

Sugar-containing beverages, processed meat, added sugars, refined grains, highly processed foods, and refined oils.

Avoid unhealthy ingredients and foods

- **Added sugar:** candies, soda, table sugar, and ice cream
- **Refined grains:** pasta made of refined wheat, white bread, etc.
- **Refined Oils:** cottonseed oil, canola oil, and soybean oil
- **Trans fats:** It is found in margarine along with other processed foods
- **Processed meat:** Hot dogs, processed sausages

- **Highly processed foods:** Anything labeled with "diet" or "low-fat" or appears to be made in an industrial unit

Whenever you go shopping, you must read the list of ingredients and avoid buying anything that contains the above components.

Foods you can comfortably eat

A typical Mediterranean diet can consist of any amount of these foods since they are healthy and unprocessed.

- **Vegetables**

Broccoli, tomatoes, kale, onions, spinach, cauliflower, Brussels sprouts, carrots, cucumbers, etc

- **Fruits**

Bananas, apples, oranges, strawberries, pears, grapes, dates, melons, figs, peaches, etc

- **Seeds and nuts**

Walnuts, almonds, Macadamia nuts, cashews, hazelnuts, pumpkin seeds, and sunflower seeds

- **Legumes**

Peas, Beans, lentils, pulses, chickpeas, and peanuts

- **Tubers**

Sweet potatoes, potatoes, yams, and turnips, etc

- **Whole grains**

Brown rice, whole oats, rye, corn, barley, buckwheat, whole grain pasta and bread, and whole wheat

- **Seafood and fish**

Sardines, salmon, trout, tuna, oysters, mackerel, shrimp, clams, mussels, crab

- **Poultry**

Turkey, Chicken, duck, and more

- **Eggs**

Duck, chicken, and quail eggs

- **Dairy**

Greek yogurt, yogurt, cheese

- **Spices and herbs**

Basil, garlic, mint, sage, rosemary, nutmeg, pepper, cinnamon, etc

- **Healthy fats**

Olives, Extra virgin olive oil, avocado oil, and avocados

In short, you must remember a one-liner: food with a single ingredient is always good for health, be it in any diet.

What you should drink

The healthiest beverage in the Mediterranean diet or any other diet for that matter is water. You cannot underestimate the importance of water in the Mediterranean diet. If you still want something else to drink, you can take one glass of red wine per day. However, if you are an alcoholic or you have any other health condition, you must avoid wine.

You can also take tea and coffee, but you must avoid beverages sweetened with sugar such as fruit juices. They contain very high amount of sugar.

A few facts worth noting

The foods that should be included in the Mediterranean diet is a matter of controversy because of the different kinds of foods and cultures of various countries. The Mediterranean diet includes a lot of plant- based foods and a low amount of animal- based foods. However, seafood and fish are recommended twice a week. You should not forget that you are going to eat significantly high calories. Therefore, make sure that you include moderate exercise in your regime. Moreover, Mediterranean culture also requires you to enjoy your life and share your meals.

A sample Mediterranean menu for a week

If you are going to start the Mediterranean diet, you can begin with the help of this sample Mediterranean menu for a week. Later, you can develop your own menu according to your suitability.

Monday

- Breakfast: Greek yogurt along with oats and strawberries.
- Lunch: A sandwich of whole grain bread with vegetables.
- Dinner: A tuna salad with a dressing of olive oil. A piece of any fruit for dessert.

Tuesday

- Breakfast: Oatmeal and raisins
- Lunch: The leftover tuna salad from last night.
- Dinner: Salad with olives, feta cheese, and tomatoes.

Wednesday

- Breakfast: Omelet with tomatoes, onions, and veggies. A piece of any fruit for dessert.
- Lunch: Whole grain sandwich along with fresh veggies and cheese.
- Dinner: Cook a Mediterranean lasagna

Thursday

- Breakfast: Yogurt with nuts and sliced fruits.

- Lunch: Consume the leftover lasagna that you did not eat last night.
- Dinner: Broiled salmon with vegetables and brown rice.

Friday
- Breakfast: Vegetables and eggs fried in some olive oil.
- Lunch: Greek yogurt with nuts, strawberries, and oats.
- Dinner: Grilled lamb along with baked potatoes and salad.

Saturday
- Breakfast: Oatmeal with nuts, raisins, and one apple.
- Lunch: Whole grain bread sandwich with some veggies.
- Dinner: Mediterranean whole-wheat pizza, topped with olives, vegetables, and cheese.

Sunday
- Breakfast: Omelet with olives and veggies
- Lunch: The leftover whole grain Mediterranean pizza from last night
- Dinner: Grilled chicken along with potatoes and vegetables. You can take any fruit for dessert.

You are not required count your calories and track your macronutrients such as carbohydrates, fat, and protein in a the Mediterranean diet.

Healthy snacks in the Mediterranean diet

Although you will not feel hungry between the three meals of the Mediterranean diet, you can eat these snacks if you still feel like eating.

- Handful of Mediterranean nuts
- Baby carrots
- A piece of your favorite fruit
- Grapes or berries
- Slices of apple with almond butter
- Greek yogurt

How you can follow the Mediterranean diet when you are eating out

Most restaurants have foods that are Mediterranean friendly. You can eat any of these things without feeling guilty. Order something that is allowed in your diet and you are all set.

- Order seafood or fish in the main course
- If you are ordering fried food, ask the management to fry it in extra virgin olive oil.
- Order only whole grain bread and olive oil in place of butter.

CHAPTER 5

Myths About the Mediterranean Diet

Despite being a tremendously beneficial diet, the Mediterranean diet is not spared of misconceptions and myths. However, you must be aware about the myths about this beautiful diet and the facts behind it.

Myth 1: The Mediterranean diet is very expensive

Fact: If the proteins you need are derived from lentils or beans, and you stick to whole grains and plants, you will not have to spend a lot on the Mediterranean diet. In fact, this diet turns out to be cheaper than dishing up processed or packaged foods.

Myth 2: You can have as much wine as you want

Fact: Many people promote the myth that three or four glasses of wine will not do any harm since wine is healthy for the heart. However, the fact is that you must take only a moderate amount of wine. It implies women can consume one glass and men can take two glasses of wine per day. Red wine is certainly healthy for your heart, but drinking it in excess has the conflicting effect. If you drink more than two glasses in a day, it may prove very unhealthy for your heart.

Myth 3: You can eat large quantity of bread and pasta

Fact: The Mediterranean people do not eat a heaping bowl of pasta like the Americans do. In fact, pasta in the Mediterranean diet is just a side dish, the serving size of which is half a cup or one cup at the most. The rest of the food on the plate consists of vegetables, salads, fish, and a small amount of grass-fed organic meat. It may also include a slice of whole grain bread.

Myth 4: The Mediterranean diet is just about food

Fact: Food certainly makes a large part of the Mediterranean diet, but it is not the only constituent. You simply cannot ignore the way Mediterranean people lead their lives. While they sit for eating a meal, they do not watch television, or they do not eat hurriedly. They would sit down in a relaxed manner to have and share food with their friends or family. Bonding with others and eating comfortably is an important part of the Mediterranean culture.

Myth 5: You can consume any kind of vegetable oil because all of them are healthy

Fact: Oils are a complicated part of any diet. There are two kinds of vegetable oils:

- The cold-pressed traditional oils like peanut oil and extra virgin olive oil that contain high amounts of monounsaturated fats. These are extensively used in the Mediterranean diet. They are produced without using any heat or chemicals for extraction.

- Secondly, the modern oils that are processed oils such as sunflower oil, soybean oil, canola oil, corn oil, cottonseed oil, vegetable oil, and safflower oil. These oils are manufactured in factories and typically from genetically modified crops or GMOs. They use toxic solvents and high heat for the extraction of oils from seeds.

Research has established that high heat and other elements can impair the oil and convert their fatty acids into trans- fat, which is very harmful for your health. The high content of omega-6 may also imbalance the proportion of omega 3 fatty acids and omega 6 fatty acids, which is again crucial for great health.

How you can make changes to your diet the Mediterranean way

Do not feel intimidated by the contemplation of changing your way of eating according to the Mediterranean diet. You can look up to these suggestions to get started.

Do not forget the vegetables

Even a minimal plate of diced tomatoes with crushed feta cheese and a drizzling of olive oil can taste simply amazing. You can also load the thin crust, whole grain pizza with mushrooms and peppers rather than pepperoni and sausage. You can consume the maximum amount of veggies in the form of crudités platters, soups, and salads.

Modify your thinking about meat

You might be fond of red meat; you can simply cut down the portion of red meat. In addition, you can choose grass fed organic meat whenever possible to stay away from hormones, GMO feed, and antibiotics that are found in abundance in industrially bred meat. You can place small strips of free-range, organic chicken on the salad platter or put a small portion of meat with a pasta dish of whole wheat.

Do not skip breakfast

Whole grains, fruits and a fiber rich meal is the best way to begin your day and keep you pleasantly satiated for longer.

Eat seafood often

The importance of seafood in the Mediterranean diet cannot be understated. You must have any kind of seafood at least twice in a week. You can have fish such as salmon, tuna, sardines, black cod, sablefish, and herring. These fish have high amount of omega-3 fatty acids. You can also have shellfish such as clams, oysters, and mussels. They are highly beneficial for heart and brain health.

Cook vegetarian food once a week

You can pick any day of the week to skip meat. Call it 'Meatless Mondays' to go meatless for at least once a week. On your meatless day, you can cook food with whole grains, veggies, and beans. After you become habitual with one vegetarian day a week, you can do it twice a week.

Consume good fats

You must consume oils and fats that are beneficial for your body such as extra-virgin olive oil, sunflower seeds, nuts, avocados, and olives. These oils are healthy sources of fats required in the daily meals

Start enjoying dairy products

Learn to enjoy products like plain yogurt, Greek yogurt, and natural cheese. When you eat full-cream dairy products, your body accumulates less fat and you have lower obesity level. This might be the result because full fat products make you satiated quicker and keep you feel full for a long time. Therefore, you do not feel the craving to eat every 30 minutes. However, you must choose raw or organic milk whenever possible.

Be careful of your desserts

When you want to eat dessert, you can eat a piece of your favorite fruit in place of cakes, pastries, or ice creams. You can eat fruits such as fresh figs, strawberries, apples grapes.

How can you avoid the mercury contained in fish

Seafood is definitely healthy for your heart. However, you cannot ignore the fact that all shellfish and other fish contain dashes of pollutants such as the poisonous metal mercury. You can look at these guidelines to stay away from such toxic substances.

- The amount of pollutants and toxic mercury is found in more amounts in larger fish. Therefore, it is better to keep away from large fish such as shark, king mackerel swordfish, and tilefish.

- The recommended amount of seafood for most adults is 12 ounces a week or two servings of 6 ounces a week.

- Learn from your local advisories of seafood whether the fish that is supplied in your area is safe for consumption.

- Children below the age of 12 years, pregnant women, nursing mothers should eat fish or shellfish that have low amount of mercury such as canned light tuna, shrimp, salmon, catfish, and pollock. Since tuna also contains high content of mercury, you must not eat over 6 ounces of albacore tuna in a week.

CHAPTER 6

Things You Must Know About the Mediterranean Diet

The crowd supporting 'calorie is calorie' has always promoted the idea of eating more and exercising even more for the last three decades. It was not surprising that the psychological, intangible, and physical failure trailed, often companied by self-loathing and anguish.

More health conscious people have often asked these groups that if there is no difference in good and bad calories, then why they should bother about gaining fat on their body. Such inconsistencies mark out these people who love promoting esoteric and intangible messages that only some people can follow. Recently, the Mediterranean diet has become the focus of the diet world since it is not complicated at all and is easy to follow.

Keeping the matter of low-fat and calories aside, the diet world often suggests such things which confuse people and are difficult to follow.

It is impossible to count indefinable calories. Another mysterious mantra for diet is to follow the diet based on plants. The Mediterranean diet fits well with the mysterious dietary recommendations as a part of eat less, low fat food and exercise more.

The Mediterranean diet largely varies depending on the region, its people and the period of time. A true Mediterranean diet can only be followed by people living around the sea, but the scientists and diet experts have conceptualized it according to the people living in plains. A normal Mediterranean diet incorporates healthy eating and a slight inclusion of olive oil and red wine, along with other constituents characterizing the conventional cooking approach of the countries that border the Mediterranean Sea.

The majority of healthy regimes include vegetables, fruits, whole grains, and restricted unhealthy fats. Although these things about a healthy diet are tested and tried, there are differences or variations in proportions of foods that might create a difference regarding the risks of heart ailments.

A few things about the Mediterranean diet may make it difficult to follow. For instance, you may not find nut oil in America so easily, which might confuse the followers of the Mediterranean diet.

What if you are not able to control yourself?

If you go to Italy, you would often hear that you must have pasta, gelato, bread, and pizza. If you do not relish these things in Italy, your trip is not complete. However, these are not meant to be eaten on a daily basis. If you are on a tour for two weeks, it is suggested that you do not indulge in delicacies every day. Keep a couple of days off from junk food even when you are holidaying.

You can go to some other Mediterranean country to enjoy the breathtaking sights of beaches with some Campania wine. While you explore food, wine, and culture of a Mediterranean state, you must not forget the thoughts regarding nutrition and health. Even in your home country, you can eat tasty food as well as healthy food at the same time.

Gelato is just another name for ice-cream. This may not go down well with many readers, but it is true that gelato is Italy tastes more or less same as ice cream.

Even in France or Greece, you might not find many people who would suggest a traveler to think about health. When they talk about gelato, they would never mention that you can skip it if you want to. France is famous for its hospitality and they serve food with so much affection that you would not be able to refuse anything that comes on your platter. You would hardly hear about the cultural significance of Florentine Steak, bufala mozzarella, and bronzino fish.

It is fascinating to see how our mind works when we rationalize justification for poor choices of eating, particularly when they concern the culture. Culture of any community is a sensitive and sacred issue. You would notice more often that when you try to modify your food choices to gain good health, it becomes most difficult to discard eating those things that are unhealthy, but are linked to your culture. For instance, you cannot stop eating bread overnight because it has passed through hundreds of cultures. There are many other things that are deep fried in oil in many cultures and they hold significant value, especially during festivals. If you refuse such things, you invite the wrath of your family members. The elderly will often scold you saying that a piece of fried bread is not going to harm you in one day. However, they are hardly concerned what that piece of food is going to do to your months of efforts for your diet.

However, Italy is different is this regard. You would not hear many people forcing you to eat something just because you should eat it as an element of their culture. A great thing about cultural differences in Italy is that different foods give you a taste of different spices, flavors, and ways of preparation of healthy foods. In the meanwhile, ever-present bread only works as a vehicle for foods such as jam, olive oil, butter, or anything else.

Pesto sauce and salmon taste amazingly good and are a healthy way of using preparation techniques and cultural seasoning to give dressing to a healthy meal.

Food observations about the Mediterranean diet

Many studies have established that when carbohydrates are replaced with fats, overall health is improved. The Mediterranean diet consists considerably of bread, pizza, meat, fish, and pasta. You will be surprised to know that legumes are quite rare in the Mediterranean diet and even nonexistent in many Mediterranean regions. If you are in Italy, you will be served a bread basket with each meal. While the locals use only a single piece of bread to soak the oil and fat on the platter after they finish the meal, you will find many foreigners eating up the whole basket of bread as appetizer. It is interesting to see that white bread is served most of the time, in place of whole grains. However, many restaurants serve whole grain bread as well.

As stated earlier, pasta is consumed in much smaller quantity than it is eaten in America. When the Mediterranean dinner is begun, you can have a small portion of pasta. If you are not habitual to Mediterranean, you might find it difficult to have a very small segment of pasta. Tourists in France, Italy, and Greece are often seen eating large portions of pasta.

The traditional sauces of the Mediterranean diet contain meat. The conventional local appetizers also contain cured meat, tomato slices, and cheese.

Organ meat in Mediterranean diet

Organ meat is not consumed in high amounts in Mediterranean diet, but it forms a part of the regime in some countries such as Northeast Africa, which is quite close to Southern Italy. The Maasai region of Africa is famous for drinking fresh goat blood. It may sound crazy to Americans, but fresh blood is enormously dense with nutrients. Many tribes of the world drink blood for nutrients and when we discard animal blood, we must now think twice about it.

The Italians also have a blood pudding, the Swedes consume blodplättar, the English eat black pudding, the Finns consume veriohukainen - all these cuisines demonstrate the worth of blood. Moreover, now you know that consumption of blood is multicultural and is not just popular with Maasai and vampires!

The Maasai love raw blood so much that they combine it with some raw milk as well. Moreover, the Maasai people also consume raw organ meat too. The abdomen of an animal is slit and the organs are removed for raw consumption. The remaining meat cuts are treated as scraps by them, which are favoured by other cultures of the world. These scraps discarded by the nomadic groups are sold in supermarkets. The Maasai and other nomadic groups devour the organs and body parts we often jeer at. In addition, they eat these groups eat raw organs, which is nowhere in comparison to the grilled meat of muscles that Americans eat several times a week.

Why are organs eaten and the remains discarded?

You must be wondering why these people do not eat the muscle meat. The Maasai people target to optimize their foods by eating foods that have maximum nutrition and contain the highest amount of calories and vitamins. Since people living in jungles have limited access to food, they try to have maximum nutrition from minimum food. Our ancestors did the same for millions of years, even those belonging to the Mediterranean countries.

This kind of diet provides up to 5-10 times the daily recommended allowance of minerals and vitamins for

Americans. You will find high amount of minerals, vitamins, omega-3 fatty acids, etc., in this diet. When you compare this diet with a typical American diet, you will find that the majority of Americans are not able to meet the recommended criteria of vitamin, B-6, vitamin A, calcium, magnesium, and zinc.

America has the best researchers, scientists, and physicians of the world, still the country has a recommended diet that places its citizens at a situation of a diet lacking in minerals and vitamins. At the same time, we call thepeople of Africa and Southern Italy as illiterate, but they know more about the human body than any of us. They know how to feed the body, which parts of other animals they need to consume to have the best nutrition possible, while the civilized part of the world consumes scraps.

The Mediterranean diet and Mediterranean fitness

While concluding this book, it is important to discuss the fitness level of Mediterranean people. There is a difference between health and fitness, which many people do not know. Fitness implies to be able to perform a task such as fit to procreate, fit to jog in a marathon, fit to scale up a staircase, etc. Fitness, however, does not characterize health. If one is fit for something, it may even lead to deteriorated health. For instance, if you are fit for running in a marathon, you may suffer from joint pain or heartache after a few years.

Europeans walk for a significant time daily and this is not hidden from the world. This is the reason that they stay slim. Italians are also much more concerned about their health than Americans. That is why; Mediterranean diet focuses on exercising a lot while you eat a lot. Americans completely lack awareness about fitness because of their sedentary lifestyle and poor diet. When you are travelling to Mediterranean states, you will be completely ripped off by the cab drivers if you cannot walk for a mile or so. You are required to be extremely fit to stay or travel comfortably in Mediterranean places. If you adapt the Mediterranean diet completely, you get several benefits such as freedom from anxiety and stress. You can be a true Mediterranean or even semi-Mediterranean in true sense only when you adopt physical fitness into your lifestyle. Once you become habitual to walking a few miles in the morning, you will not be able to quit that regime.

CONCLUSION

Be it America or any other culture, people often use lack of diversity as justification to keep away from a healthy diet that does not consist of pasta and bread. Healthy diets contain often low amount of carbohydrates, which makes us uncomfortable with the new regime. And we always have a problem coming out from our comfort zone.

A significant amount of carbohydrates is often spoon fed to people to impart comfort. For instance, when you were sick with fever in your childhood, you must have received toast with cinnamon and sugar. If your aim was literally flavor variety and food, simply mundane pasta and bread would play a slight role.

Perhaps the finest part of following a nutrient dense diet is that it includes intense flavors, which most Americans miss out on with their regular diet. If you want to bring positive changes into your food regime, you can cook something next time that gives you more experience like that of a connoisseur. Food is not just about eating; food is at its best when you feel it and enjoy it with others.

The Mediterranean diet focuses on the idea of sharing food

and enjoying life, rather than just eating for living. Even an animal can eat to live, but we are not animals. We have been gifted with such brains that we are perfectly able to judge what is good and what is bad for us, even if we have not read or know much about it. Our body itself lets us know what should be fed to it and what not.

You must have read about organ meat in the last chapter of this book. Sometimes, you can add it to your meals to add some variety in a literal sense and reap the benefits as well. You never know you may start liking it. The Mediterranean diet uses olive oil in their most basic cuisines, but red wine is consumed with caution. Even though you might see Mediterranean people drinking red wine at lunch or dinner every day, they do it with care. No Italian is easily found drinking red wine to get high; it is just a part of a healthy meal.

In brief, the Mediterranean diet is definitely a healthy way of living, provided you follow it arduously. Since you already know that you do not have to follow any tough restrictions with this diet, you can adapt it for life. You will be surprised to see the changes in your health and the enhanced glow on your skin. That is why; you must have seen that the Mediterranean women often have a gracious glow on their faces. If you follow the diet mentioned in this book, the day is not far away when you will be grabbing praises from your peers.

Good luck for a healthy life!

www.ingramcontent.com/pod-product-compliance
Lightning Source LLC
Chambersburg PA
CBHW072139290526
45789CB00013B/1632